30 Days to

Food Freedom

LEARNING TO MANAGE
WEIGHT & EATING BEHAVIORS
WITHOUT DIETING

DEDICATION

This book is dedicated to the love of my life, Rob Solberg, who found me when I was lost, put me back together when I was broken, loved me when I was unlovable, and made me believe that I was worth fighting for.

My heart is forever yours.

CONTENTS

Introduction

If you have ever struggled with overeating and weight issues you know how it can completely take hold of your life. Not only because the food cravings and food obsession seem ever-present, but also because the burden of the extra weight can be a source of shame. It's a constant reminder of failure and our inability to control ourselves, and the burden grows with every failed attempt to lose the weight.

My struggle with weight began in the fourth grade. I loved sugar and ate it whenever I wanted to experience pleasure in the midst of a traumatic and dysfunctional childhood. When I started putting on weight, it seemed as if the whole world noticed and had something to say about it. I was teased and bullied daily by family members and school kids. I was always anticipating the next cruel comment, always aware of my abnormality. I was ashamed of my body and my lack of self-control, and I started believing the message that I was unacceptable and unworthy unless I was thin.

As the years passed I felt more and more powerless to control myself around food and I became desperate. My thoughts were full of anger and frustration; *"Why can't I just lose this weight once and for all? Why can't I stay on a diet? I don't want to look like this and I hate myself for getting here!"* Those thoughts and feelings overpowered me and always pushed me back to using food as my emotional solution, my comfort, and my temporary high; thus becoming the source of more weight gain. This was the vicious cycle of addiction. I was a full-blown food addict (although I didn't know it at the time) by my early twenties.

By the age of 22 I was obese and miserable. My life was consumed by losing (and regaining) weight, my emotions were dictated by what the scale said and by a constant awareness of my flawed body and what others must be thinking. I had grown to believe that the shell I was living in was my identity. My heart, my gifts, and my purpose in life took a backseat to my body image. I believed that I could never love myself or be loved unless I was thin.

My path to freedom began in 2010 through Celebrate Recovery, 12-step recovery program that had just come to my church. I had no idea that food addiction was a real issue or that the power to control one's eating without recovery is almost non-existent for those, like me, who have a propensity to use food as a drug. I felt relief and hope that there may be an answer. Could I finally be free from this?

I fully invested myself in the Celebrate Recovery program and also began attending another twelve-step food recovery program in 2013. It was hard work, but as a result of working the steps I started losing weight and I was *not* dieting. I felt so free! I focused first on losing the "fat in my head" and as I worked on the inner me the outer me started to release extra weight. I wasn't a slave to a diet or gimmick, I was actually transforming; becoming a new person. Or maybe I was just discovering the person that was always there, the one who got caught up in addiction and lost in the darkness that had claimed her God-given identity. For the first time I believed God was willing and able to help me overcome my food issues, so I started letting Him take the lead. It was new to me to share this struggle with Him and to believe that He could and *would* help.

My 70-pound weight loss was only one of the gifts I received through this recovery journey. My mind and my heart have also been transformed, and my life is filled with more joy, more peace, and more purpose than I ever thought possible. These are the things that I could never see while I was blinded by my obsession with food and my weight. And these are the gifts that are waiting there for you, too, if you're willing to start on this journey.

Recovery is about progress, not perfection, and I'll be the first to admit that my recovery has been far from perfect. I still struggle and I still have weight I would like to lose to be healthier (*not* to be thin). But because my recovery calls for a daily dependence and communication with God, my Father, I don't have to do it under my own power. There is now an acceptance of where I am today, with peace and patience instead of fear and urgency. God reminds me to look at how far I have come, and to stay out of living in a future that's not here yet.

I was so inspired by the freedom I'd finally found after decades of agony fighting it on my own that I wanted to share my story and the recovery tools and concepts I'd learned and developed along the way. I became a Certified Nutritional Consultant so I could help those who struggle with the same issues I do, offering encouragement, accountability and education on food choices and eating behaviors. I am not a medical professional or a mental health professional, but I am a specialist in food addiction having lived and studied both sides of it for most of my life.

If you can identify with any part of my story, this book is for you! It offers a 30-day guide to *permanent life change* based on the success and experience I have had in my own recovery. It is designed to address the various ways that unhealthy dependence on food can manifest itself in our lives, and it's written for people at all levels, from the occasional emotional eater to the hardcore binge eater, and everything in between.

If you're ready to make a change in your life this book will help! How do you use it? Just read one day at a time, and don't rush through it. Set aside 20-30 minutes of quiet time each day to go through the lesson. Each day includes one or more tools you can incorporate into your journey, action steps, inspirational quotes, and a relevant scripture to help you address the all-important spiritual side of recovery.

If you want to learn more or have any questions please visit my blog at DebSolbergHealth.com.

I pray that this 30-day journey brings about real life change and healing for you and helps you move closer to the purpose and plan that God has for you!

Day 1

NOTHING CHANGES
IF NOTHING CHANGES

Today is a new day, an opportunity for you to step onto a new path. The path to freedom unfolds one day at a time, one step at a time, one decision at a time. There is no better time than today to give yourself the gift of health and wholeness!

You can be free from shame, from negative thoughts, and from the guilt and anger that you carry throughout the day due to poor decisions about food and about your health. You don't have to overeat when you feel emotion-you can change that starting today. And with patience and diligence, you will be free from the burden of extra weight you carry as a result of your compulsion to use food as anything other than fuel and energy.

Are you ready for real, permanent change? Are you willing to do what it takes to achieve it? Because nothing changes if nothing changes!

Today's Action Steps

1. Make a list of all of the ways you have used food in unhealthy ways.

2. Now write down the physical and emotional results of those actions.

3. Now write down the ways it has affected those around you.

4. What are some of the things that would be different in your life if you were free from the thoughts and feelings that come from being controlled by negative body image and by the obsession with food? Write about it.

5. Do you believe that God wants a whole and purposeful life for you? Meditate on the following scripture and pray that He will give you everything you need to change, just for today.

Today's Scripture

"I waited patiently for the Lord, and he inclined to me, and heard my cry. He brought me out of a horrible pit, out of the miry clay, and set my feet upon a rock, and established my steps!"
—Psalm 40: 1-2

Today's Inspiration

"Man often becomes what he believes himself to be. If I keep on saying to myself that I cannot do a certain thing, it is possible that I may end by really becoming incapable of doing it. On the contrary,

if I have the belief that I can do it, I shall surely acquire the capacity to do it even if I may not have it at the beginning."
—Mahatma Gandhi

Day 2

ELIMINATING BINGE FOODS

When I first heard my compulsive overeating issues described as an "allergy of the body" I was intrigued. One of the definitions of the word *allergy* is, "an abnormal reaction of the body to a previously encountered allergen".

The phrase that jumped out at me in this definition was "abnormal reaction". Did I have an abnormal reaction to certain types of foods? You better believe it. Specifically sugar and white flour foods. If I consume them, the result is always the same: intense cravings for more. And more and more.

Ask anyone who has had issues with bingeing on certain types of foods and they will tell you that it feels beyond their control to stop. This reaction is not something that can be muscled through with willpower. For a food addict, this allergy is very real.

This is why it was so important for me to start identifying my allergens. These were the triggers that resulted in binges, obsession, depression and extra weight. Eliminating these foods was the only choice I had if I wanted to experience freedom.

Abstaining from my trigger foods (desserts, breads, white pastas, sugar cereals, refined carbohydrates) was *the single most important thing I did* to become free from overeating. It was also the biggest factor in weight loss for me and for so many others I know who have felt defeated by emotional and compulsive overeating.

The practice of abstinence is not always easy, and that's why we commit to doing it just for today. *This is not a diet.* This is a life change for health, energy, and freedom from the weight in your mind and body.

Today's Action Steps
1. Make a list of all foods that you can't eat just one of.
2. Make a list of the foods that cause you to overeat when you are stressed or emotional.
3. Eliminate these foods from your diet. Since sugar is usually the main culprit, make sure you read the list of ingredients on the packaging and stay away from foods that contain added sugar (bread, crackers, even ketchup can be culprits). You may experience a withdrawal period from 3-10 days with possible headaches, mood swings and mental fatigue. Hang in there. You will feel amazing on the other side!

Today's Scripture

"Do you not know that your bodies are temples of the Holy Spirit, who is in you, whom you have received from God? You are not your own."

—1 Corinthians 6:19

Today's Inspiration

"If you want what you do not have, you must do what you have not done."

—Dave Ramsey

Day 3

THE ESSENTIAL FOOD PLAN

A daily food plan is absolutely critical in my recovery from food addiction. When I am tempted to just "wing it" because I am too busy or too distracted to take the time to plan, I remember that my meal plan is my battle plan. Its what keeps me free from acting out compulsively around food.

My food plan is important for many reasons:

- It keeps me aware that I have the propensity to overeat and it helps me stay within boundaries.
- It prevents me from "grazing" all day. When I avoid the oral fixation of grazing in between meals, the obsession and the cravings eventually go away. I am replacing the unwanted behavior with a healthy behavior.

- If in-between-meal cravings occur, my food plan gives me the opportunity to look to other solutions to conquer them, finding what methods work for me, making it easier to get through them.
- My food plan tells me when to eat, instead of my feelings.
- It gives me the freedom to say "no" to all other food decisions throughout the day because I know ahead of time those decisions are usually unhealthy and compulsive.

My food plan is my safety and security from that first compulsive bite. Sometimes I will need to be flexible because my schedule can change and life can change. So I adjust accordingly, focusing on freedom.

Today's Action Step
Plan three healthy, moderately portioned meals and one snack (as necessary) per day. Make sure you are including protein and a vegetable with each meal.

Today's Scripture
"The plans of the diligent lead surely to abundance, but everyone who is hasty comes only to poverty."
—Proverbs 21:5

Today's Inspiration
"By failing to prepare, you are preparing to fail."
—Benjamin Franklin

Day 4

JOURNAL THERAPY

When I take the time to honestly process my feelings by getting them out of my head and onto paper (or computer screen) something magical happens. I am another step further along in learning how to face my fear, discomfort and pain without using food to push down my emotions. When I practice this daily I start to connect the dots. Things start making sense that never did before. My secrets come out of the darkness and into the light where they can heal. I get to know myself better and start to identify the "life cues" that bring on the feelings that cause me to run to food. My writing can even help solve problems and resolve conflict in my life. The best part is I can be unabashedly honest since my journal is for my eyes only.

I also use my journal to write out my prayers to God. This helps me stay focused on what I'm writing so I am not as likely to be distracted as I am when I pray without a pen. And over time I can look back at my journal entries to see God's amazing provision and power, and how He has answered my prayers and given me hope for another day!

Today's Action Steps
1. Start a journal to use for daily prayer, reflection, and working through feelings and cravings.
2. Whenever you feel like eating compulsively, go to your journal and write about it. You will be amazed at how the more you write, the less you crave.

Today's Scripture
"Call to me, and I will answer you and tell you great and mighty things which you do not know."
—Jeremiah 33:3

Today's Inspiration
"Journal writing is a voyage to the interior."
—Christina Baldwin

Day 5

MOVE!

A common myth believed by many newcomers to exercise is that in order to for it to be effective, physical activity has to be a long, strenuous, sweat-drenched endeavor. I couldn't disagree more! Although there is nothing wrong with pushing your body to higher fitness levels, spending hours every week killing yourself at a gym is not realistic or sustainable for most people, especially someone just starting out on his or her personal fitness journey. Exercise needs to be both enjoyable and achievable in order to be sustainable.

Move in accordance with your current fitness level, move so you enjoy it, but the important thing is to *move*! Don't make it harder than it needs to be, but don't cheat yourself either. As long as you are putting the time in, make the most of it. Start by walking 4-5 days a week for 30 minutes. In time you can add to or replace your walking with other activities you may want to try. You will be amazed at how much more energy and peace you will have each day!

Why is moving your body so important? Because your body was designed to move. Regular exercise not only benefits you physically, it has tremendous emotional and psychological advantages as well. When you elevate your heart rate, powerful mood-boosting chemicals are released into your brain that help improve your self-esteem, enhance your mood, improve your memory and mental functioning, and decrease your stress. Conversely, study after study shows that living a sedentary lifestyle will shorten your lifespan, diminish your quality of life, and increase the likelihood that you will suffer from a chronic disease. Bottom line: there is no better (or simpler) solution than exercise when it comes to fighting depression, anxiety, immune system problems, low energy, sleep issues, negative eating behaviors and obesity-related diseases.

Yes, it might take some sacrifice. But if you want to find that freedom, you need to make the time for it, even when you don't feel like it. And if you do, I promise you will never regret it. In fact, if you stick with it, it will eventually become a habit and you will actually start enjoying it.

Today's Action Steps
1. Take a 30-minute walk today. How about right now?
2. Set aside 30 minutes at least 4 times each week for a physical activity that you enjoy. Put it in your calendar and commit to it.
3. As your body adapts and gets more fit, challenge yourself to new activities and new fitness levels.

Today's Scripture

"I can do all thing through Christ who gives me strength."
—Philippians 4:13

Today's Inspiration

"One of the greatest moments in life is realizing that two weeks ago your body couldn't do what it just did."
—Anonymous

Day 6

DAILY BATTLE PLAN

It's unsettling but true; my food addiction is always waiting for me. While I am minding my own business, it's preparing to take me down by "doing pushups in the hallway", as they say in recovery. So our job is to be prepared. We need to stay a step ahead of it by making sure we're ready to do battle with it and anticipating its next move. This act of preparation is a very powerful tool in our fight for our freedom.

Here are some ways to stay a step ahead and grow stronger and wiser in the process:

SURVEY THE DAY
Evaluate your day for potential compulsive eating triggers. Is your day set up for possible stress? Will you be crazy busy? Will you be in contact with people who test your nerves? Is there a situation or

relationship you will be walking into that has caused you to binge or have strong cravings in the past? Don't go into these situations blind and unarmed. Take action now and plan how you are going to handle these situations ahead of time. Knowing they're there is half the battle. Commit to facing them without food.

FOOD PREP DAY

Take some time to plan meals for the week. Grocery shopping, veggie chopping, storing and cooking healthy foods will set you up for absolute success! It also allows you to include healthy choices in your food plan each day, making sure you're well nourished and feeling energized.

RESTAURANTS

There is nothing wrong with eating out, but making the wrong choice on the menu can easily turn into regret because unplanned choices can lead to bingeing. Again, preparation is key. Make your food choices *before* you go. Almost all restaurants have online menus. It might seem a bit rigid at first, but in the end you'll find it freeing! All it takes is one bad decision. That first bite of something you ordered compulsively can throw you off track and invite the shame and self-loathing back into your mind space.

WRITING

There is nothing like being completely honest about your deepest feelings when no one else will see them. When those thoughts and feelings get out into the light they begin to lose their grip on us. Even though we don't always see the direct connections, these are the same feelings we often try to avoid and numb with food. This is why unexpressed feelings can lead to cravings; it mimics old behavior patterns.

Today's Action Step

Take a few minutes today to ensure that you are setting yourself up for success by preparation and planning using the key points above.

Today's Scripture

"Therefore, prepare your minds for action, keep sober in spirit, fix your hope completely on the grace to be brought to you at the revelation of Jesus Christ."
—1 Peter 1:13

Today's Inspiration

"There are no secrets to success. It is the result of preparation, hard work, and learning from failure."
—Colin Powell

Day 7

PRAY FOR HELP

I've found that one of the most important tools I need in order to be free from emotional overeating is willingness. My willpower is only temporary and I've come to recognize that I cannot be willing enough on my own to be successful today. So I ask God to give me the will and the ability to stay on this path to freedom. I ask Him for the strength that I don't have on my own to live today free from the clutches of my affliction. And there is nothing more He wants for me. Because when I am free from the daily consequences of "drugging myself" I am able to connect with Him so much more and He is able to fill the void in my soul that I had been trying to fill with food.

What does willingness look like to me? Here are some questions I ask myself:

- Am I willing to ask God to help me with food decisions when I am tempted to take the first bite that might lead me off this path of physical, mental and spiritual restoration?
- Am I willing to stay aware of my eating behaviors today?
- Am I willing to plan my meals today?
- Am I willing to abstain from the foods that I use as a drug?
- Am I willing to feel discomfort in order to win the battles I encounter today?
- Am I willing to pray and journal my feelings today?
- Am I willing to put myself first and not eat carelessly to satisfy or "love" others?
- Am I willing to face the fear that encompasses going without certain foods?
- Am I willing to accept where I am today and focus on freedom, not on my weight?
- Am I willing to believe that God will help me through all of this if I ask Him? After all, He desires this freedom for me just as much as I do!

Today's Action Step

Pray today for the willingness and the ability to do what it takes to be free from the control of food and negative eating behaviors.

Today's Scripture

"You, God, are my God, earnestly I seek you; I thirst for you, my whole being longs for you, in a dry and parched land where there is no water."

—Psalm 63:1

Today's Inspiration

"This also means that God won't let you use weakness as an excuse for not doing what He's asking you to do."

—Rick Warren

Day 8

CRAVINGS

No matter how far along you are in your recovery from compulsive overeating, you will, at some point, experience a craving to eat something that has given you trouble in the past. Or you'll be tempted to eat a food that is on your trigger list, hoping to reintroduce it to your diet. I have done both and I can tell you this experimentation is definitely not worth it! It is exactly like an alcoholic saying he or she will only have one drink. All it does is bring on more cravings, which eventually lead to another binge and all the misery that comes with it. Remember, cravings are not commands! You *do* have a choice. Don't let your craving tell you what to do.

Here are some guidelines that will help you work your way through those cravings and stop them in their tracks, so you can stay on track.

- Sit down and write about how you feel when you're eating clean and not being a slave to food.
- Remember that going back to old habits is a choice. You can choose to return to a life of unhappy emotional eating binges, weight gain, anger, and frustration. OR you can choose to do without that first bite.
- Accept this craving as natural. The temptation, and this moment, will pass.
- Remember every time you say "no" to compulsive overeating it makes it easier for you to do it the next time. You're building your "no muscle"!
- Remember that food won't make any bad situation better.
- Think about how good it will feel to wake up tomorrow knowing you didn't binge or eat compulsively today.
- Remember the trouble and misery you experienced as a result of giving in to your last craving. How did that work out for you?
- If the craving persists, eat a serving of raw fruit or vegetables to stop it from going any further.

Remember to stay in the moment. All you need to do is the next right thing. This is especially true when it comes to frustration with the number on the scale. Your weight loss may be happening even now, and it *will* happen eventually as long as you're staying within your food plan and away from trigger foods. Remember, the number on the scale will definitely *not* go the way you want if you eat over it.

Today's Action Step

Should you experience cravings for any binge foods today, use the guidelines discussed in this chapter.

Today's Scripture

"For since He Himself was tempted in that which He has suffered, He is able to come to the aid of those who are tempted."
—Hebrews 2:18

Today's Inspiration

"True comfort is to be found in the balance of sanity of abstinence. So deep and pure is this comfort that it is well worth whatever trouble or pain I might have to pass through to attain it."
—Voices of Recovery, Overeaters Anonymous

Day 9

THE SCALE

Let's face it; the vast majority of us aren't motivated to get free from compulsive overeating because we are happy with our weight. As a matter of fact, in my recovery group there is a saying, "Come for the vanity, stay for the sanity."

For most of us, the number on the scale seems to make or break us. It can dictate our moods, take up too much of our mind space, and remain an obstacle in our path to freedom from obsession with food and body image. Therefore, we need to be very careful to use the scale only as an accountability tool and a practical measure of our progress to get to a healthier weight.

Since I have an eating disorder I know that even when I am abstinent, I can still find sneaky ways to be compulsive; larger food portions, sneaking bites while cooking, an extra snack here and there, etc. So first, I need to acknowledge the fact that the scale can actually be a helpful tool by keeping me informed about my health and telling me the truth about whether or not I am overeating. My weight should not be the focus of my recovery, but it *is* a symptom of my disease. And if that symptom is flaring up it means my disease is not being managed properly. The trick is to learn how to weigh ourselves without it becoming an obsession, like it has with every diet we've been on.

I have found (and experts agree) that for a person with eating issues and anxiety with weighing themselves, a weigh-in once per month is appropriate. Step on the scale one time, then put it away! Resist the temptation to weigh yourself again. If the number is creeping up (beyond a couple pounds) consider making changes to your food plan. Review your process; are you consuming things you haven't planned? If you need to weigh and measure your food portions, do it for accountability.

The most important thing is to be patient. Each day should be a celebration of how much you are changing on the inside. Trust that the outside will follow in time. Remember, your weight is only a barometer of your how your food plan is working for you. Don't give it any more power than that!

Today's Action Step
Decide on a day and how often you will weigh yourself to gauge how well your food plan is working. Then stick to it. No more, no less.

Today's Scripture

"Therefore, since we are surrounded by such a great cloud of witnesses, let us throw off everything that hinders and the sin that so easily entangles. And let us run with perseverance the race marked out for us."

—Hebrews 12:1

Today's Inspiration

"Losing a pound isn't necessarily a reward. Being healthy and feeling good about yourself is the reward."

—Nancy Peterson

Day 10

THE NEED FOR GOD TODAY

I recently heard a pastor say, "Sin is a legitimate need met in an illegitimate way." He went on to use overeating as an example of this truth. Looking back through my years of using food as a drug, I could completely relate to this. Overeating was an illegitimate way to fill my deepest longings and satisfy my legitimate needs. Food was what my flesh wanted and what I went running to for comfort. In short, it was my God.

Through recovery I've learned that *all* of our needs can be satisfied by God. He created us and knows what we need even better than we do. He formed us, He loves us, He values our existence and He has plans for our lives. Growing and sustaining our relationship with Him is the only way to true wholeness and peace. He is the only comfort that we need and the only One who can fill our deepest longings.

In my many years of addiction I reached for what my flesh was craving, thereby separating myself from God and pushing Him away. As a consequence, because of the cycle of self-hatred, guilt, anger and over-indulgence that occupied my mind, I couldn't grow emotionally or spiritually. Trying to heal my loneliness, sadness, and pain with food was like pouring water on a drowning woman. It drove me deeper into my pain and darkness. Every time I chose not to reach out to God and instead reached out to food, I was putting my trust in something fleeting and weak. Every time I trusted food for my peace and comfort, it failed me. Every. Single. Time.

This is why daily prayer and meditation are so important. And its why it's so vital that we "pray in the moment" when the battle gets tough. Praying for willingness to stay "clean", asking for guidance, and then letting go of our own self-will (which is what got us here in the first place!) will help us develop the insight and intuition to do the next right thing. God is faithful. He will fill those empty spaces and longings within us if we stay in relationship with Him daily. And eventually we will be at a place where reaching out for food isn't our default anymore. We will reach out to the loving arms of our Father!

Today's Action Steps
1.   Pause and include God in your daily decisions.
2.   Realize the importance of surrendering to what He wants for you instead of what you want.
3.   Trust that He knows what you need and what will always sustain you.

Today's Scripture

"'For I know the plans I have for you' declares the LORD, plans to prosper you and not to harm you, plans to give you hope and a future.'"

—Jeremiah 29:11

Today's Inspiration

"Much of your pain is self-chosen. It is the bitter potion by which the physician within you heals your sick self."

—Khalil Gibran

Day 11

INSIDE OUT CHANGE

In some ways, this path to freedom that starts from the inside out can mimic a diet, because we're avoiding certain foods, planning meals and measuring portions. How many diets have we been on in the past and how did that work out for us? More importantly, how is this path any different? There are actually a number of significant differences between a diet and true recovery from food addiction or emotional overeating:

A Diet...

- Has a beginning and an end
- Gives the illusion of controlling the outcome, when in reality you can only control the process
- Only changes the body, and this is usually just temporary. The obsession with food and eating remains

- Puts the focus on the "symptom" (the weight) rather than the "disease" (the unhealthy thoughts and behaviors that led to the weight)
- Measures success by a number on the scale rather then true life change
- Is powered by our limited and temporary willpower
- Is unsustainable for life

Recovery from the inside out...

- Is ongoing and sustainable for life
- Brings positive daily change to the whole person; mind, body and soul
- Puts the focus on freedom from our obsession with food, body image and compulsive eating—the weight comes off naturally as a byproduct
- Measures success by the absence of damaging behaviors, thoughts and actions
- Offers less restrictive food options; we're free to enjoy healthy, normal portions of whatever foods aren't triggers that cause us to binge
- Is powered by God as we learn to surrender to Him daily
- Brings more patience and serenity since the number on the scale isn't the primary focus

As we're regularly making choices that lead us further away from our "former life", our eyes are opened and we begin to see the differences between how we used to manage our health and how we are doing it now. Our weight loss efforts in the past have always backfired because our excess weight is just an outward symptom of what is going on inside of us. Once we identify the thoughts and subsequent behaviors that are causing us to carry the extra weight we can change those behaviors and finally start to release the extra weight, gaining health on the inside *and* the outside! As the saying goes, "Focus on the weight and lose your recovery. Focus on your recovery and lose the weight".

Today's Action Steps
1.   Think about and list the ways you are changing on the inside since you started on your path to freedom.
2.   Write about how this is different from your previous weight loss attempts.

Today's Scripture
"Don't copy the behavior and customs of this world, but let God transform you into a new person by changing the way you think. Then you will learn to know God's will for you, which is good and pleasing and perfect will."
—Romans 12:2

Today's Inspiration
"The scale can only give you a numerical reflection of your relationship with gravity. That's it. It cannot measure beauty, talent, purpose, life force, possibility, strength, or love. Don't give the scale more power than it has earned."
—Steve Maraboli

Day 12

ACCEPTANCE

Acceptance, as we use the word in recovery, does not mean that you approve of something; it simply means that you acknowledge, "it is what it is". In order to experience victory and end each day successfully we need to learn to accept our circumstances as they are, not as we would have them. It's when we *don't* accept our circumstances that feelings become uncomfortable, stressful and we're tempted to eat compulsively.

The act of accepting our current circumstances in the recovery process will snap our minds into awareness. Acceptance provides us with comfort and peace during times of temptation and helps to build our confidence.

Put into practice the following each day:

- Tell yourself out loud that you accept yourself unconditionally as you are today.
- Accept the truth that God is with you. He wants you to let go of your damaging behaviors so He can take over. He will be your help when you ask Him and let Him.
- Accept the fact that you have trouble controlling your food impulses and that it is causing damage in your life.
- Accept the fact that just one compulsive bite could draw you into a binge and/or more cravings.
- Accept the fact that food won't make *any* situation better.
- Accept that you will experience occasional and temporary discomfort in the form of cravings, raw feelings and the urge to eat between planned meals.
- Accept that recovery is about progress, not perfection.
- Accept that your body will respond to your new way of eating and start shedding the extra weight in it's own time.

And most importantly accept each day of recovery as it's own, one day at a time.

Today's Action Steps

1. List anything or anyone in your life that you are in conflict with, angry with, or worried about.
2. If any of these circumstances are beyond your control, accept that this is just the way life is right now. Surrender the people or circumstances to God and trust that He is in control and will work things out in His timing and in His own way.

Today's Scripture

"And we know that in all things God works for the good of those who love him, who have been called according to his purpose."
—Romans 8:28

Today's Inspiration

"Acceptance doesn't mean resignation; it means understanding that something is what it is and that there's got to be a way through it."
—Michael J Fox

Day 13

STOPPING THE INSANITY

As a child, I remember that a sweet treat would always bring me comfort when I was feeling things I didn't want to feel. That treat represented more than just an occasional indulgence; it was an escape from a reality I didn't like and couldn't control. Slowly but surely the occasional treat grew into many treats, and over time the importance of those treats grew for me as well.

Since it was bringing me a pleasure that temporarily numbed my pain, I wanted more of it. Just like an alcoholic or drug addict, I started needing more and more of those treats to be satisfied. My quest for comfort resulted in bigger and more frequent binges. The pain of feeling full to the point of nausea and bloating, the shame of gaining weight (then dieting, then gaining weight again), the feeling of being out of control, the purging and starving myself out of fear, the outbursts of anger, and the self-loathing were not enough to stop

44

me from reaching for that first bite again the very next day. This was the definition of insanity playing out my life; I was doing the same thing over and over and expecting different results.

Over time, through recovery, we can learn now to hit our knees in prayer, reach for our journal, or talk to a trusted friend when we start to feel those uncomfortable feelings. We come to realize overeating will not cure our loneliness, make our anger and worry go away, or resolve an argument with a family member or friend. Only God can do those things. So today choose to let Him help you with your difficult feelings and circumstances, because He already chose you as His own. Today choose sanity!

Today's Action Steps
1. Divide a piece of paper into two columns.
2. In the first column describe how the overuse of food affects you physically and emotionally.
3. In the second column write about how you feel when you have had a day of mindful, abstinent eating.
4. Post this on your refrigerator and read it when you have the urge to binge.

Today's Scripture
"Come to Me, all you who labor and are heavy laden, and I will give you rest."
—Matthew 11:28

Today's Inspiration

"Insanity: Doing the same thing over and over and expecting different results."

—Albert Einstein

Day 14

PUTTING YOURSELF ON PAUSE

One of the major factors that contributed to my years of binge eating was the fact that I was really good at intentionally "checking out" before and during an episode of stuffing my face with food. I didn't want to stop to think about what I was doing because I was afraid to face reality without the comfort and pleasure of the food. I was afraid if I stopped and thought about it I might see the reality of my situation. I knew deep down that I was mistreating myself, but the sick part of me didn't care. I wanted what I wanted in that moment, consequences be damned. And it turned out the consequences were that I would remain stuck in a vicious cycle of eating, guilt and shame for years.

If we want to replace our blind eating behaviors with the intentional behavior of choosing abstinence and responsible eating we have to stay aware any time we're making food decisions. When we feel ourselves gravitating toward old habits (which is normal) we need to learn to pause before we make a destructive decision we will surely regret. Some of the things we can ask ourselves in that moment include:

- Will this make my situation better?
- Will this make me feel as good as I do when I'm abstinent?
- Will this make me stronger in my recovery?
- Will the freedom and peace I have now be compromised?
- Will this be a setback and cause a relapse in my recovery?
- How will I feel about this after I've eaten it? Or tomorrow morning?

It's amazing how well this "pause method" steers your mind back into the reality that, yes, this decision will be harmful to you. Has a binge or a compulsive eating decision ever come without consequences for you? Has it ever made things better for you in the long run? There is something about consistently exercising the "no muscle" that gives us the strength and confidence to move on into another day of freedom!

Today's Action Step
Practice mindfulness when it comes to each food decision. If the food isn't in your meal plan for the day, pause, pray and put it back!

Today's Scripture
"Be still, and know that I am God."
—Psalm 46:10

Today's Inspiration

"Have patience. All things are difficult before they come easy."
—Saadi

Day 15

MISTAKES & MISSTEPS

If there is one thing I've learned during my recovery from food addiction its that mistakes and missteps *will* happen. I am a perfectionist through and through and sometimes my program just does not go the way I intended it to. More often than not this is due to a poor decision on my part.

We always need to remember that this recovery journey is about progress, not perfection. No misstep on it's own has the power to pull us back into the food. We get to choose how to respond our mistakes. Do we throw in the towel? Or do we get up off the ground, dust ourselves off, and continue on our journey? Ultimately the choice is ours, and only one of those two options leads to freedom.

That said, it's a lot easier to *prevent* a relapse than to climb out of one. So what do you do when you find you're making poor decisions and have allowed your "all or nothing" attitude to take over? Here are a few tools you can use.

WRITE ABOUT IT

What circumstances led you to overeat? What can you do next time in these same circumstances to prevent it? Be careful not to overanalyze. Sometimes the "whys" can pull us into too much self-condemnation. Write a prayer asking God to clear your mind of it and give you the peace not to condemn and shame yourself, but to move on.

ACCEPT IT

Shake hands with it and realize you are not perfect. Recognize that food can be as powerful as a drug when used as a temporary emotional solution. Keep in mind that it's not your fault that you have this problem, but you *are* accountable—to yourself and the people who love you—to pursue the solution.

FORGIVE

Forgive yourself for the mistake and don't give it any more power over you. Remember, you are on a path to freedom! Don't give in to the temptation to punish yourself by starving, skipping meals or over-exercising. You are leaving those habits and patterns behind. They never worked for you in the past, and they certainly won't work now.

POSITIVE ACTION

No matter how frustrated you are with yourself, think of one positive, healthy thing you could do for yourself or someone else today that will make you happy, then do it. This will help you to stay positive and hopeful and learn how to move on with grace.

Today's Action Steps
Use this page if you have had a slip or a setback in your journey to freedom. Review and practice these key points to ensure this was just a stumble, not a relapse!

Today's Scripture
"I have said these things to you, that in me you may have peace. In the world you will have tribulation. But take heart; I have overcome the world."
—John 16:33

Today's Inspiration
"If we are to experience recovery from compulsive overeating, we will have to repeat, day after day the actions that have already brought us so much healing."
—Overeaters Anonymous

Day 16

DON'T GIVE UP

Recently I came across a very inspiring quote:

"Don't give up on what you want for what you want right now."

This beautifully sums up the thought processes, decisions and actions that encompass our food choices and where they will lead, every single day. After reading that quote I made two lists in my journal:

1. What do I want?
   - To be peaceful each morning when I get up because I was abstinent the day before.
   - To be free from any obsession with food; free from craving it, missing it, and flirting with thoughts of indulgence of foods that are on my abstinence list.

- To be free from regret and self-loathing because of bad choices.
- For my clothes at my smaller, healthier size to fit, or to fit into a smaller size I have never been before that is healthy and sustainable
- To have the courage to pursue the plans God has for me because I'm not in a "food fog."

2. What do I want right now, in the moment, when I'm tempted to overeat or indulge a craving with a trigger food?
- I want a piece of food for the momentary, fleeting pleasure of eating.

Do you see the cruel trade off? When you feel like taking that first compulsive bite, or when you catch yourself thinking that all of this effort isn't worth it because you're missing your favorite foods, re-read the quote above.

Today's Action Steps
1. Post the quote above on your refrigerator or pantry as a reminder that perseverance is life!
2. List the reasons you will continue to practice abstinence, stay on your meal plan, exercise, and make nutritious food choices today.

Today's Scripture
"No temptation has overtaken you that is not common to man. God is faithful, and he will not let you be tempted beyond your ability, but with the temptation He will provide a way of escape, that you may be able to endure it."
—1 Corinthians 10:13

Today's Inspiration

"Patience and perseverance have a magical effect before which difficulties disappear and obstacles vanish."

—John Quincy Adams

Day 17

CELEBRATE THE WINS

I'm a recovering perfectionist. So 99% of things in any situation could be going right, but I'm drawn to the 1% that could be "better". The 1% screams at me to give it all the attention while I ignore the wonderful 99%. This self-critical behavior is due to a combination of my natural (controlling) personality and the consequences of a chaotic childhood.

Through food recovery I've learned how valuable it is to celebrate the wins. Even if I feel like I've failed miserably in any aspect—as a parent, in my job, in my relationships or my recovery—I know there is something worthy of celebrating. I may be struggling with my eating today, but at least I've set my feet on the road to recovery. That's a major accomplishment on it's own. I may not be where I want to be, be at least I'm not where I used to be.

No matter how we feel about ourselves, or how someone tries to make us feel, we need to stay aware of our thoughts and practice the habit of replacing negative thoughts with the positive. We need to remember daily to "think about what we are thinking about". This discipline helps prevent our thinking from leading us into unhappiness, anger and stress, which can lead to another binge.

If we're constantly beating ourselves up we steal our own hope and joy. When we clutter our minds with negativity and start believing the lie that we're not worthy unless we do everything right we're setting ourselves on a collision course with unhappiness. On the other hand, when we accept our imperfect selves as works-in-progress and humbly acknowledge the small victories we open ourselves up for growth. We *will* struggle and we *will* fall. But falling is not failing! And the only way we can fail after a fall is by refusing to get back up. Each time we choose to get back up, we grow a little more perseverance, hope, and mental toughness in the process.

Today's Action Steps
1. Start writing your accomplishments at the end of every journal entry, no matter how small you think they are.
2. Whenever you feel negativity creep up in your mind throughout the day, remind yourself how far you have come.

Today's Scripture
"Finally, brothers and sisters, whatever is true, whatever is noble, whatever is right, whatever is pure, whatever is lovely, whatever is admirable—if anything is excellent or praiseworthy—think about such things."

—Philippians 4:8

Today's Inspiration
"Whether you think you can or you can't, you're right."
—Henry Ford

Day 18

STAY IN TODAY

Once in awhile I find my mind wandering into thoughts I have no business thinking. I worry about the future, fear scenarios that haven't happened (and probably never will), and ask myself the nagging question that almost all recovering addicts ask at some point. "How am I going to keep this up for the rest of my life?" Our tendency to try to "live in tomorrow" really stems from a need for control.

When I feel this thinking start to overtake me I have a couple of simple phrases that I will literally speak out loud; "Stay right here", or, "Keep your head where your feet are." I then take a mental inventory of where I am in the present moment, realizing I need to "come back" and stay in today and not wander into the future where my mind wants to imagine doom, gloom and failure. This present moment is a gift and it's all that is real. Worrying about tomorrow will not change a single thing about it. Our focus should be on living today to it's fullest. We can rest in the knowledge that God is in control and He is taking care of our today and our tomorrow too.

Today's Action Steps
1. Stay in the present moment.
2. Whenever you start to fear or worry about the future, remember that those things have nothing to do with the present moment.
3. Read today's scripture twice!

Today's Scripture
"Therefore I tell you, do not worry about your life, what you will eat or drink; or about your body, what you will wear. Is not life more than food, and the body more than clothes? Look at the birds of the air; they do not sow or reap or store away in barns, and yet your heavenly Father feeds them. Are you not much more valuable than they? Can any one of you by worrying add a single hour to your life? And why do you worry about clothes? See how the flowers of the field grow. They do not labor or spin. Yet I tell you that not even Solomon in all his splendor was dressed like one of these. If that is how God clothes the grass of the field, which is here today and tomorrow is thrown into the fire, will he not much more clothe you—you of little faith? So do not worry, saying, 'What shall we eat?' or 'What shall we drink?' or 'What shall we wear?' For the pagans run after all these things, and your heavenly Father knows that you need them. But seek first his kingdom and his righteousness, and all these things will be given to you as well. Therefore do not worry about tomorrow, for tomorrow will worry about itself. Each day has enough trouble of its own."
—Matthew 6:25-34

Today's Inspiration

"Worry does not empty tomorrow of it's troubles, it empties today of its strength."

—Corrie Ten Boom

Day 19

FEELING FEELINGS

Our feelings can be a challenge. They can invite pain, shame and memories that we would rather avoid. In order to buffer ourselves from these uncomfortable feelings, and because we can feel so out of control about what's happening on the inside, we often find ourselves acting out on the outside in an area where we *think* we have some control: food. But, of course, this behavior ends up creating even more negative feelings, which, in turn, we follow and act upon. This perpetual cycle creates discourse in our relationships and keeps us unhappy and burdened with negativity.

By eliminating our trigger foods and maintaining abstinence over them we are breaking that cycle and making room for God to step in and help manage those feelings. Our negative emotions start to subside because we are no longer feeding them by using our "drug". God is doing for us what we could not do on our own. We can now face our feelings and be less fearful about them. We find we have more wisdom and the awareness to pause and examine our emotions. And we develop the ability to discard those feelings that are unhealthy and unworthy of reacting to. Remember: feelings aren't facts. They don't always have to be followed!

Most importantly, our line of communication to God is no longer distorted because He is now in control of our lives, rather than the food or our emotions. So we spend less time being tossed around by waves of emotion, and instead, through Him, we start to enjoy lives of stability and serenity.

Today's Action Steps
1. Stay aware of feelings today and pay attention to how you react to them.
2. Remember you can choose not to act out when it comes to negative feelings. Instead of acting on them, write about them in your journal.

Today's Scripture
"So as a man thinketh in his heart, so is he."
—Proverbs 23:7

Today's Inspiration
"Abstinence is a lifeboat. Stay in the lifeboat."
—Overeaters Anonymous

Day 20

THE LIGHT OF TRUTH

Most of us who are (or have been) overweight have been ridiculed because of our body size. For me, this created deep shame. I was conditioned to believe I did not fit in and I was not important or valuable because of the way I looked. The negative daily messages I received did serious damage to my self-esteem and I started to believe I didn't deserve anything good in my life. At least not until I was thin. I lived a lot of my life believing those lies and as a result I lost my true identity and character. "Fat" and "unacceptable" ruled my being and stole away the true me that God created.

As we do the work of recovering from food issues, practicing daily abstinence and time with God, we begin to see things in the light of truth, rather than through the distorted lens of our compulsion with food. As a result, layer after layer of hurt, judgment and shame is peeled back and replaced by peaceful acceptance and understanding.

The accusing inner voice fades away allowing us to hear the *real* inner voice of God speaking truth to us. The dots start to connect. The road that led to our issues with food becomes clearer and we gain insight into the reasons behind some of our character defects. This is so important because it allows us to recognize, to forgive, to heal, and ultimately to leave the past in the past.

The journey to recovery and health is hard work, but it is so worth it. It's truly transforming, inside and out!

Today's Action Steps

1. Do you remember a time in your past when someone hurt you with words? Write about how it affected you and the damage it may have caused in your life.

2. Now write a letter to that person, defending your honor. (Don't worry; you don't need to send it. This is an exercise for *you*.) Tell them why it hurt and tell them the truth about how God feels about you. Use a bible if you need to, there are many verses that describe His love for you!

Today's Scripture

"For you formed my inward parts; you knitted me together in my mother's womb. I praise you, for I am fearfully and wonderfully made. Wonderful are your works; my soul knows it very well. My frame was not hidden from you, when I was being made in secret, intricately woven in the depths of the earth. Your eyes saw my unformed substance; in your book were written, every one of them, the days that were formed for me, when as yet there was none of them."

—Psalm 139: 13-16

Today's Inspiration

"Your time is limited, so don't waste it living someone else's life. Don't be trapped by dogma, which is living with the results of other people's thinking. Don't let the noise of other's opinions drown out your own inner voice. And most important, have the courage to follow your heart and intuition."

—Steve Jobs

Day 21

FEAR OF HUNGER

I have a rule: The food I pack in my lunch bag or put on my plate is my complete and final meal and it stays in accordance with my food plan for that day. The amount of food I portion out is what I eat and nothing more. Since I am a compulsive overeater these boundaries are vital for my success. It's not about calorie restriction, it's about controlling my compulsive eating behavior, which can include things like going for seconds, eating while I'm cooking, and unplanned snacking.

There have been days—even well into my recovery—where I've noticed I get anxious about these boundaries. Is this amount of food going to be enough? What if I get hungry later? Shouldn't I have a backup plan? Normal eaters don't obsess like this. Normal eaters "go with the flow" when it comes to eating. It's just fuel for the body; they will eat again at some point, no big deal.

Pre-recovery, I ate all day long. I had to have something to pacify me because most of the time I was a mess inside. Grazing all day in between meals had become a way of life for me, a deeply rooted habit. My "three meal-a-day" (and sometimes a snack) food plan is one of the most powerful tools I've found to break myself out of that bad habit. It was a challenge at first, but now it feels amazing.

These days I don't think about going hungry between meals. I've actually adopted the "no big deal" attitude about food that I used to think was impossible for me. The good habit has been put into practice long enough to replace the bad. And when those anxious feelings do creep in, I'm prepared with some simple self-talk and a prayer. For example:

SELF-TALK
"You will eat again at some point. Hunger is just a feeling and it's OK to feel it. It won't kill you."

PRAYER
"Lord, let this be enough."

COMMON SENSE
If my meals are well-balanced, nutrient dense, and moderately portioned, they *will* be enough!

Today's Action Steps
   1.   Ask yourself, "What is the worst thing that could happen if I'm hungry for awhile?" Write about it.
   2.   Engage the principles above when you feel the fear of "going without".

3.   Whenever you feel hungry between meals, embrace it, and know that, although it may be a little uncomfortable, it is normal.

Today's Scripture
"Cast your cares on the LORD and he will sustain you; he will never let the righteous be shaken."
—Psalm 55:22

Today's Inspiration
"Let your food plan tell you when to eat, not your feelings."
—Unknown

Day 22

THE ILLUSION OF CONTROL

For a lot of us, the most common triggers for food binges are worry and stress about things we have no control over. Sometimes we even invent imaginary scenarios to worry about, scenarios that have not happened and probably never will! This used to be a way of life for me. When people or circumstances got out of my "control" and things didn't go the way I wanted or expected the anxiety would send me right to the food.

I had fooled myself into thinking my eating was something I could control. And the food *did* comfort me...for a minute. But always, without fail, my bingeing became one more thing for me to worry about. It always did more damage than I intended or expected. And it always left me feeling (you guessed it) out of control. Which, of course, just set me up for yet another episode of bingeing. And so the cycle continued.

Fortunately I learned a simple truth along the way that helped me break out of that cycle and address my tendency to worry and control: the only thing I have control over is me. Specifically that means my actions and my attitudes. The idea that I can control anything or anyone else is an illusion. God is in control of the universe and I need to let Him have control of my life as well.

When faced with any circumstance in life where it would be fruitless to worry or try to control it (which, by the way, is *every* circumstance in life), practice letting go and trusting God with the outcome. Stay out of His way and trust that He knows what is best for you. It's not always easy, believe me. Sometimes circumstances are painful and so hard to let go of! But trust God. He will never fail you.

Today's Action Steps
1. Make a list of the things you worry about in life.
2. Go through the list and ask yourself which ones you have full control over.
3. Circle the ones you do not have control over and write, "God will take care of this" next to it.
4. Pray and trust that He will.
5. Go back and look at the list in a few weeks and be in awe of His provision!

Today's Scripture
"Have I not commanded you? Be strong and courageous, do not be afraid or discouraged, for the Lord your God will be with you wherever you go."
—Joshua 1:9

Today's Inspiration
"I trust that no matter what happens in my life today, picking up the food will not take away the pain or make me feel better."
—Voices of Recovery

Day 23

THE MENTAL & EMOTIONAL BATTLE

Our preoccupation with food not only manifests itself physically in the form of cravings, it also shows up in the form of mental obsession. As a matter of fact, our thinking is what gets us into the most trouble.

We start out feeling strong, making promises to ourselves for real change, and relying on our willpower to stay away from the bad foods and eating behaviors. But at some point our mind will start telling us it's okay to go back to some of those foods and behaviors in moderation. The thoughts in our mind may sound something like this:

One bite is no big deal. I've been doing so well so I deserve a small reward. Maybe I don't have a problem with this specific food anymore.

For most compulsive overeaters like me, our minds can deceive us at a moment's notice if we're not careful. Just when we think we have control and we're standing strong we get tempted to take a bite of something we know was a trigger food for us in the past. And if we give in to the temptation, which seems so tiny in the moment, we will inevitably lose ground in the battle for our peace of mind, our healthier body, and our self-confidence.

Because we've conditioned ourselves to believe that food is the solution to our uncomfortable feelings and emotions, our willpower will never be enough. Sooner or later willpower fades. It always does. It's like a Law of the Universe. And once our willpower fades we will start to seek that old "solution" again to satisfy our legitimate need for physical or emotional comfort. How many times have you, like me, lost weight, then lost your will power and gained the weight back?

This is why the "recovery of the mind" approach is so important. Life never stops making emotional demands of us. We have to find a way to live where we aren't responding to those demands with food, but rather in healthy ways. Prayer, meditation, journaling, and talking with someone we trust are healthy ways to find comfort when our emotions cry out and we start to think maybe we can use food "just this once".

Remember, your thoughts and your emotions can be deceptive and can lead you down the path of compulsive overeating. The healthier your mind is, the less it will try to trick you into believing you can control the foods and behaviors that have worked against you time and time again. So keep practicing healthy ways to process the feelings and emotions that can lead to unhealthy decisions, and your mind will be less likely to talk you into them!

Today's Action Steps

1. Revisit your binge food list from Day 1. As you look at each item, remember the times and the emotions surrounding the overeating of those foods.
2. Reflect on the emotions you feel now that you don't eat them anymore. What has changed in your life? Write about it.

Today's Scripture

"If you think you are standing strong, be careful not to fall."
—1 Corinthians 10:12

Today's Inspiration

"Our happiness depends on the habit of mind we cultivate."
—Norman Vincent Peale

Day 24

REST

Each day our efforts to stay aware and focused on our recovery from compulsive food behaviors require that we bring our best game. With each good decision we are rewiring our brains to actually *think* before we *do*. This can be draining, especially when we're new to recovery. That's why our recovery has to include learning how to rest, conserve our energy, and avoid wasting it on things that aren't relevant to our progress.

Getting plenty of sleep is essential because tiredness can be a trigger to overeat and cause us to want to "throw in the towel". Sleep is when our body is doing its best work; repairing cells, restoring cognitive function, and renewing us for the day ahead. Too little sleep can hamper our metabolism and it can actually contribute to weight gain.

When we're tired our body is telling us it needs rest. So instead of staying up watching TV, reading, tackling a chore, or worrying about things we can't control, we need to just sleep. All of those other things will rob us of much needed rest today, which will make recovery much more challenging for us tomorrow.

Maybe, like me, you feel a need to be productive until the last minute of the day. But considering the amazing work the body does while we sleep, I'd say that "sleep productivity" wins every time!

Today's Action Step
Decide on a regular sleep schedule and make it a point to adhere to it every night. In time you will feel more energized and well rested. You'll also find it easier to fall asleep at night and wake up feeling good in the morning.

Today's Scripture
"The Lord is my shepherd, I lack nothing. He makes me lie down in green pastures, He leads me beside quiet waters, he refreshes my soul."
—Psalm 23:1-3

Today's Inspiration
"It is a common experience that a problem difficult at night is resolved in the morning after the committee of sleep has worked on it."
—John Steinbeck

Day 25

KEEPING IT SIMPLE

Food is fuel, plain and simple. It's used to sustain, build, and heal our bodies. But we have complicated things so much by using it as a drug or an emotional crutch that we are now suffering the consequences. When we're in our addictive or compulsive behaviors our minds are full of emotional and mental turmoil; worry, shame, fear, obsession about our weight, guilt, body image issues. It's chaos! But it doesn't need to be that way. The more we simplify our lives, the more effective we become.

The first step in keeping it simple is abstinence from the trigger foods that draw us into unnecessary battles. Remember, if it's not an option, it's not a problem! The best (and simplest) solution is to forgo the extra food we're thinking about, which is risking an all-out binge and setback in our program. Problem solved.

Also, our meal plan simplifies our lives and frees us from our preoccupation with food. Plan your three meals, record it, and then forget about food and focus on the opportunities of the day! It may take a little bit of intentional planning up front, but compared to how muddled and messy our lives are when we were bingeing, it's a no-brainer!

I used to think keeping things simple, measured and planned would be a restriction on my freedom and I would resent it But it has turned out to be just the opposite! The freedom I've found through this process goes to show just how convoluted and chaotic my life was before recovery, and it reminds me that I wouldn't want to go back for anything!

Today's Action Steps
1. Write three reasons why it's better and simpler for you to forgo that extra food, rather than give in to it.
2. Review your meal plan and list of trigger foods and remind yourself to keep it simple.

Today's Scripture
"For God is not a God of confusion but of peace".
—Corinthians 14:33

Today's Inspiration
"Life is really simple, but we insist on making it complicated."
—Confucius

Day 26

VIGILANCE

Maintaining abstinence and staying on our food plan can be a challenge when life pulls us out of our routine and structure. Vacations, weekends, holidays, illness, and other unexpected events can become big obstacles to our recovery. During these times it can take every ounce of prayer, strength and awareness to stay abstinent. Our recovery doesn't take a holiday or vacation just because we do!

After these events pass, the sigh of relief or "letdown" we feel can be a danger as well. Having made it successfully through a period of temptation or a difficult situation can trick us into believing we're safe and can let our guard down. Or we may start to feel we deserve a reward for the hard work we put in. Don't fall for these traps!

Compromising your abstinence by taking that first compulsive bite won't serve as a reward for all your hard work, it will *undo* all your hard work. We need to be careful not to fool ourselves into thinking that just because we overcame some big battles we are now safe. In fact, the small ones (the letdowns) are just as powerful and just as capable of doing major damage to our recovery.

When you're feeling that nagging, gnawing craving to comfort yourself in any situation, remember that it's not up to you to carry the heavy load. That job belongs to God, who acts on your behalf. Pray, ask for strength to do the next right thing, and then let go and let Him take over the fight!

Today's Action Step
Make sure you are building a battle plan not only for events like holidays, vacations, parties, etc., but also for the days following those events (the letdown). Anticipate you might want to indulge and crave food during these times as well.

Today's Scripture
"Stay alert! Watch out for your great enemy, the devil. He prowls around like a roaring lion, looking for someone to devour."
—1 Peter 5:8

Today's Inspiration
"The price of freedom is eternal vigilance."
—Thomas Jefferson

Day 27

IT'S OKAY TO THROW IT AWAY

Have you ever popped a piece of food in your mouth only to realize you didn't like it or didn't even want to eat it, but then you ended up eating it anyway because you felt you "had" to or it would go to waste? Or maybe it was so good that, even though you didn't need it, you wanted to eat it anyway? What we are really deciding in those moments is that the morsel of food or the momentary bit of taste is more valuable to us than our own physical and mental well-being. We're putting our peace and our recovery in jeopardy for no good reason.

One of the ways to break this temptation is to prepare only the servings you need for a meal and nothing more. When you're feeling hungry remember that your feelings are always bigger than your stomach. Those feelings often tell you that you need a lot more food to be satisfied than you really do. This is why it's important not to wait too long in between meals, and to eat at the same time every day.

When preparing food, focus on preparing enough to satisfy your body, not your feelings. If you portion out a moderate, nutrient-dense serving and eat slowly you will be satisfied every time. If you find there is food left over when you're done preparing the meal, immediately store it for later. Or if there's not enough to be saved, immediately throw it away. Same thing if you find you're satisfied before your plate is empty; store the extra food immediately or throw it away. It's always better to toss out a small amount of food than to overeat compulsively and experience the consequences.

These may seem like minor details, but remember, we are forming new patterns of behavior in our relationship with food. Commit to taking these small steps and you'll begin to create a future for yourself where food has no more power over you!

Today's Action Steps
1. Pay attention to the "full factor" during your daily meals. Listen for your body to tell you it is no longer hungry.
2. As soon as you get this cue, stop eating.
3. If you still have food left over, simply store it or throw it away. Don't finish it all.

Today's Scripture
"For life is more than food, and the body more than clothing."
—Luke 12:23

Today's Inspiration

"Take care of your body. It's the only place you have to live."
—Jim Rohn

Day 28

SLOW & STEADY WINS THE RACE

As long as we keep trying, there are no failures in recovery. It takes some of us longer than others to catch on and find our way to freedom from compulsive overeating and bingeing. But no matter how slow the successes are, if you're still trying, you have not failed. In fact, the only way to fail in your recovery is to give up.

So be patient with yourself, trust the process and don't become discouraged. Galatians 6:9 tells us, "Let us not become weary in doing good, for at the proper time we will reap a harvest if we do not give up."

We spend years and years developing an unhealthy relationship to food. So don't be surprised if it takes weeks or months of experimenting and working at recovery before you're able to find abstinence and stick with it. You *will* have victories along the way.

Celebrate them! Before long you'll notice that food doesn't bring you as much of that temporary satisfaction as it did before. You'll discover moments of freedom, which are really small tastes of the larger freedom that awaits you on this journey. Know that pursuing this path to freedom is the only way for us to live a whole, free life, and it's worth every bit of patience and perseverance we can muster.

As far as weight loss, I know it can be easy to become discouraged if you're finding it's coming off too slowly or not at all. It helps to remember that through this process we're not just releasing weight from our bodies, we are also learning a new way of life and losing the unhealthy weight in our minds! Unlike diets, weight loss is not our only measurement of success. In fact, our spiritual and emotional growth is even more rewarding than the weight loss, which, by the way, *will* happen eventually. This is where it helps to take our eyes off the big mountain in front of us, and instead focus on doing the next right thing. Take it one step at a time, one day at a time. If you don't give up I promise one day you will find you have conquered that mountain!

Today's Action Steps
1. List all of the ways you are changing on the inside.
2. Think about the negative behaviors you have replaced with the positive.
3. Let the way this feels sink in and be your daily objective, not your weight. The weight will follow. But the more you focus on it, the greater the chance you will return to your old behaviors.

Today's Scripture

"We are hard pressed on every side, but not crushed; perplexed, but not in despair; persecuted, but not abandoned; struck down, but not destroyed."

—2 Corinthians 4:8-12

Today's Inspiration

"Never, never, never give up."

—Winston Churchill

Day 29

GRATITUDE

There are some days I wake up and notice my attitude is already set to "ungrateful mode". I feel crabby and anxious and immediately gravitate toward the negative, anticipating the hurdles of my day and how I will need to tackle them. I basically decide my day is going to be difficult before my feet even hit the floor!

My brain defaults to that setting more times than I care to admit. But the difference now (and my saving grace) is the awareness that I am doing it. Sooner or later during one of my negative, crabby thoughts I'll stop, take notice of what I'm thinking, and immediately pursue an attitude change. And the single most powerful tool I've found in changing my attitude is gratitude.

Being grateful turns my attitude around almost immediately. I simply stop and thank God for every blessing and every trial in my life at that moment. I thank Him because I know the blessings are from Him, and I know He will give me the help I need for the trials and show me victory through them. Many times I will go to my journal and write a list of all the things I'm grateful for in my life. As I write I can feel my anxiety, burden and complaints fading away. I become aware of the beautiful things around me, the gifts I've been given, and I thank Him because I know I've done nothing to deserve it!

Today's Action Steps

1. Write a list of all things you are grateful for today.
2. Practice this frequently to purge any negativity, self-pity and resentment you may be feeling.

Today's Scripture

"Do not be anxious about anything, but in every situation, by prayer and petition, with thanksgiving, present your requests to God."
—Philippians 4:6

Today's Inspiration

"Gratitude is the healthiest of all human emotions. The more you express gratitude for what you have, the more likely you will have even more to express gratitude for."
—Zig Ziglar

Day 30

GOING BACK TO NORMAL EATING

Compulsive overeating is a manageable behavior, but it is not curable. This means there is a 0% chance that those of us who struggle with this issue will ever be able to successfully partake in "normal" eating for any length of time. That is, if you define normal eating as, "eating as much as you want of whatever food you want whenever you want it without negative consequences."

Once we accept the fact that our lives will go back to being unmanageable if we return to our old "normal" eating habits, we will stop trying to go back to those habits, which caused our misery in the first place. Through this act of acceptance we come to realize that our old eating habits were actually very abnormal!

Through recovery we find a new normal for our eating, a *healthy* normal. Under this new, healthy normal we will find that we can eat as much as we want, because our compulsive desire to overeat is under control. We can eat whatever we want, because our bodies and our minds now want healthy foods. And we can eat whenever we want, because our desire to remain free and at peace means we only want to eat when it's time to eat.

As you're on your journey of recovery prepare yourself for the new normal ahead. Accept the fact that when you reach your desired weight you will still need to live by your food plan and avoid your personal trigger foods. But this new normal is going to be glorious compared to the old normal you're leaving behind!

Today's Action Steps

1. Go back through the previous 30 days and make a list of the daily lessons that resonated with you the most.
2. What was the most surprising thing you learned about yourself?
3. What was the biggest change you made in your relationship with food?
4. What's the biggest lie you stopped believing?
5. Reflect on the ways you've changed in last 30 days and thank God for your victories.

Today's Scripture

"And the God of all grace, who called you to his eternal glory in Christ, after you have suffered a little while, will himself restore you and make you strong, firm and steadfast."

—1 Peter 5:10

Today's Inspiration

"Even as your body betrays you, your mind denies it."

— Sara Gruen

ABOUT THE AUTHOR

Debra Solberg is a Certified Nutritional Consultant, author and speaker specializing in emotional eating, food addiction and body image issues. Her own battle with obesity and sugar addiction have given her a passion to help others achieve victory over what can seem like an impossible undertaking. Debra works regularly as a Health Coach and speaker, and is an advocate and participant in a 12- step program for dealing with negative food behaviors. She is a certified Indoor Cycling Instructor, a worship leader, and a professional singer with the band Dust & Daisies. Last (but really first), she is a lover of Jesus Christ, a happily married woman and a proud mom of two amazing and gifted girls.

www.DebSolbergHealth.com
www.DustAndDaisies.com

www.ingramcontent.com/pod-product-compliance
Lightning Source LLC
Chambersburg PA
CBHW060153290526
45789CB00003B/1025